Dr. Cohen Simple Diet Cookbook

How To Make 10 Simple Smoothies

(Smoothies And Recipes)

Dr. Cohen.

Table Of Contents

Introduction To Smoothies.

Smoothies are a delicious and healthy way to add more fruits and vegetables to your diet. They are packed with essential vitamins, minerals, and antioxidants, making them an excellent option for a nutritious breakfast, a post-workout snack, or an anytime refreshment.

The best part about smoothies is that they are incredibly versatile and can be customized to suit your taste preferences and dietary requirements. You can use a wide range of fruits and vegetables, such as berries, spinach, kale, banana, and avocado, along with nuts, seeds, and dairy or non-dairy milk.

To make a smoothie, you will need a blender or a food processor, along with fresh ingredients of your choice. It is important to choose high-quality ingredients that are fresh and free from any contaminants. You can opt for fresh or frozen fruits and vegetables, depending on their availability and your taste preference.

When making a smoothie, you can adjust the consistency to your liking by adding more or less liquid. You can use water, coconut water, milk, or any non-dairy milk, such as almond, soy, or oat milk. You can also add some sweeteners, such as honey or maple syrup, if you prefer a sweeter taste.

One of the best things about smoothies is that they are incredibly easy and quick to make. All you need to do is add your ingredients to a blender and blend until smooth. You can also add ice cubes or frozen fruits to make your smoothie more refreshing.

In this guide, you will find a variety of smoothie recipes that are easy to make and delicious to taste. Whether you are looking for a green smoothie, a fruity smoothie, or a protein-packed smoothie, we have got you covered. So, grab your blender and get ready to enjoy the goodness of smoothies

Chapter 1: Benefits Of Smoothie

Smoothies are a popular drink that can provide many health and nutritive benefits. Here are some of the key benefits of consuming smoothies:

Nutrient-Dense: Smoothies can be a convenient way to pack in a variety of nutrients into one drink. They can be made with a variety of fruits, vegetables, and other ingredients like nuts, seeds, and protein powders, providing a wide range of vitamins, minerals, and other beneficial compounds.

Hydration: Smoothies can be a great way to stay hydrated, especially if you use a liquid base like water or coconut water. Staying hydrated is essential for maintaining overall health and can help with digestion, circulation, and more.

Digestive Health: Smoothies can also support digestive health by providing fiber and probiotics. Fiber can help keep your digestive system regular and healthy, while probiotics can support the growth of beneficial gut bacteria.

Immune Support: Smoothies can be rich in vitamins and minerals that support immune health, such as vitamin C, vitamin A, zinc, and iron. Consuming these nutrients can help strengthen the immune system, reducing the risk of infections and illnesses.

Energy Boost: Smoothies can be a great way to boost energy levels naturally. They can be made with ingredients like bananas, berries, and leafy greens that provide a steady source of energy without the crash that can come from consuming sugar-laden beverages.

Weight Management: Smoothies can be a healthy and satisfying way to support weight management goals. They can be made with low-calorie ingredients like leafy greens, cucumber, and celery, which can help keep you feeling full and satisfied while reducing overall calorie intake.

Skin Health: Smoothies can also support skin health by providing antioxidants, vitamins, and minerals that help reduce inflammation and support collagen production. Ingredients like berries, citrus fruits, and leafy greens are particularly beneficial for skin health.

Chapter 2: Smoothie-Making Tips and Techniques

Smoothies are an excellent way to pack in essential nutrients and stay hydrated. Whether you're a seasoned smoothie pro or a newbie, here are some tips and techniques to help you make delicious and healthy smoothies every time.

Choose the Right Blender: The blender you use can make or break your smoothie-making experience. A high-powered blender is recommended as it can quickly and easily blend even the toughest ingredients like kale or frozen berries. Look for a blender with a powerful motor, sharp blades, and a large capacity.

Use Frozen Fruit: Frozen fruit makes your smoothie thicker and creamier while also giving it a colder and more refreshing texture. It's also an excellent way to use up fruits that are about to go bad. Simply freeze your fruits in advance or buy pre-frozen fruits from the store.

Add Greens: Greens like spinach, kale, and collard greens are packed with vitamins and minerals and are an excellent way to add nutrients to your smoothie. Add a handful or two to your smoothie for an extra nutritional boost.

Mix Liquid and Solid Ingredients: Always add your liquid ingredients first, followed by the solid ingredients. This helps to prevent your blender from getting stuck or jammed. It also ensures that your smoothie is blended evenly.

Experiment with Different Liquids: Instead of using only milk or water, try adding different liquids like coconut water, almond milk, or even green tea to your smoothie. These liquids can add flavor and extra nutrients to your smoothie.

Use the Right Amount of Liquid: Use the right amount of liquid to achieve your desired smoothie consistency. If you prefer a thicker smoothie, use less liquid. If you prefer a thinner consistency, add more liquid.

Add a Sweetener: Adding a natural sweetener like honey, maple syrup, or dates can enhance the flavor of your smoothie without adding any refined sugar. Adjust the amount of sweetener to your liking.

Blend in Stages: Blend your smoothie in stages to ensure that everything is evenly mixed. Start with the liquid, then add the softest ingredients like fruits and greens, followed by harder ingredients like ice or nuts.

Customize to Your Taste: Experiment with different ingredients and customize your smoothie to your taste preference. Add protein powder, nut butter, or superfoods like chia seeds or acai berries for an extra nutritional boost.

Serve and Enjoy: Once your smoothie is blended, pour it into a glass and enjoy immediately. If you have any leftovers, store them in the fridge for up to 24 hours.

Chapter 3: Necessary Equipment for Making Smoothies

Making smoothies requires some basic equipment to ensure that you can create a smooth and consistent blend. Here are the necessary equipment you'll need to make smoothies:

Blender: A blender is the most important piece of equipment you'll need for making smoothies. Look for a blender with a high wattage motor and a good quality blade that can handle frozen fruit, ice, and tough greens like kale.

Measuring cups and spoons: Measuring cups and spoons are necessary to ensure that you're adding the right amount of ingredients to your smoothies.

Cutting board and knife: A cutting board and knife are essential for cutting and preparing your fruits and vegetables before blending.

Mason jars or glasses: Mason jars or glasses are great for serving your smoothies. Look for jars or glasses that can hold at least 12 ounces of liquid.

Straws: Straws make it easier to enjoy your smoothie, and they can also be used to stir the ingredients.

Optional equipment:

Ice cube trays: Ice cube trays are useful if you prefer to use ice cubes in your smoothies.

Nut milk bag: A nut milk bag is useful if you prefer to make your own nut milk or strain your smoothie to remove any pulp or seeds.

Food processor: A food processor can be useful if you're making smoothies with tough ingredients like nuts, dates, or seeds.

Immersion blender: An immersion blender is a handheld blender that can be used to blend ingredients directly in a glass or jar.

Chapter 4: 10 Healthy Smoothies

1 Carrot Cake:

Carrot cake smoothie is a delicious and nutritious drink that's perfect for breakfast or as a snack. It's made with fresh carrots, banana, yogurt, and spices to create a creamy, sweet, and spicy flavor reminiscent of classic carrot cake. Here's a recipe that serves 2:

Ingredients:

2 medium carrots, peeled and chopped

1 ripe banana, peeled and sliced

1 cup plain Greek yogurt

1/2 cup unsweetened almond milk

1/4 cup rolled oats

1 tsp vanilla extract

1 tsp ground cinnamon

1/4 tsp ground nutmeg

1/4 tsp ground ginger

2 tbsp maple syrup (optional)

Directions:

Add the chopped carrots, sliced banana, yogurt, almond milk, rolled oats, vanilla extract, cinnamon, nutmeg, and ginger to a blender.

Blend on high speed until smooth and creamy, about 1-2 minutes. If the mixture is too thick, add more almond milk as needed.

Taste the smoothie and adjust the sweetness as desired with maple syrup.

Pour the smoothie into two glasses and serve immediately.

Nutritional Value:

This carrot cake smoothie is a great source of vitamins, minerals, and fiber. Here's a breakdown of the nutritional value per serving:

Calories: 211

Total Fat: 4g

Saturated Fat: 1g

Cholesterol: 5mg

Sodium: 130mg

Total Carbohydrates: 34g

Dietary Fiber: 5g

Sugars: 18g

Protein: 13g

Tips:

For a vegan version, substitute the Greek yogurt with a non-dairy yogurt of your choice, such as coconut or almond milk yogurt.

Use a high-speed blender to ensure a smooth and creamy texture

Add more or less almond milk to adjust the thickness of the smoothie to your liking.

If you prefer a sweeter smoothie, you can use a sweetened vanilla yogurt or add more maple syrup.

Add a handful of ice cubes to the blender for a refreshing and chilled smoothie.

2. Avocado Sunrise Smoothie

Description:

This smoothie is a delicious and healthy way to start your day! It's packed with nutritious ingredients like avocado, banana, orange juice, and Greek yogurt, and the vibrant colors make it a visually stunning drink as well.

Ingredients:

1 ripe avocado, pitted and peeled

1 banana, peeled

1 cup orange juice

1/2 cup plain Greek yogurt

1 tsp honey (optional)

1 cup ice cubes

Measurements:

1 ripe avocado, pitted and peeled

1 banana, peeled

1 cup orange juice

1/2 cup plain Greek yogurt

1 tsp honey (optional)

1 cup ice cubes

Directions:

Add the avocado, banana, orange juice, Greek yogurt, and honey (if using) to a blender.

Blend on high speed until the mixture is smooth and creamy.

Add the ice cubes to the blender and continue blending until the ice is completely crushed and the mixture is well combined.

Pour the smoothie into a tall glass and enjoy!

Nutritional Value:

This smoothie is loaded with healthy nutrients, including fiber, potassium, vitamin C, and healthy fats from the avocado. Here's the approximate nutritional breakdown per serving:

Calories: 375

Fat: 19g

Carbohydrates: 50g

Fiber: 11g

Sugar: 28g

Protein: 8g

Tips:

Make sure your avocado and banana are ripe for the best texture and flavor.

If you don't have Greek yogurt, you can use regular yogurt instead.

Add more or less ice to adjust the consistency of the smoothie to your liking.

If you want to make the smoothie even healthier, you can add a handful of spinach or kale to the blender for extra greens.

3. Banana Nut bread

Banana nut bread smoothie is a delicious and healthy drink that is perfect for breakfast, snack or dessert. This smoothie is a blend of ripe bananas, walnuts, almond milk, and spices that give it the taste and aroma of a freshly baked banana nut bread. Here is a detailed recipe to help you make this delicious smoothie at home.

Ingredients:

2 ripe bananas, peeled and sliced

1 cup unsweetened almond milk

1/4 cup walnuts, chopped

1/4 tsp ground cinnamon

1/4 tsp ground nutmeg

1/4 tsp vanilla extract

1 tsp honey (optional)

Directions:

In a blender, add the sliced bananas, chopped walnuts, almond milk, cinnamon, nutmeg, vanilla extract, and honey (if using).

Blend all the ingredients until smooth and creamy.

If the smoothie is too thick, you can add more almond milk to adjust the consistency.

Taste the smoothie and adjust the sweetness by adding more honey if needed.

Pour the smoothie into glasses and serve chilled.

Nutritional Information:

This banana nut bread smoothie recipe makes two servings. Each serving contains approximately:

180 calories

8g fat

26g carbohydrates

4g fiber

4g protein

Tips:

You can use any type of nut milk instead of almond milk.

If you want a thicker smoothie, you can add a frozen banana instead of a fresh one.

You can substitute the walnuts with any other nuts of your choice, such as pecans or almonds.

To make this smoothie vegan, you can omit the honey or use a vegan sweetener like agave nectar.

For an extra boost of protein, you can add a scoop of vanilla protein powder to the smoothie.

4. Pina colada smoothie

Description:

This Piña Colada Smoothie recipe is a refreshing and delicious tropical drink that's perfect for a warm day. It combines the flavors of pineapple and coconut, and can be made in just a few minutes with a blender.

Ingredients:

1 cup frozen pineapple chunks

1 banana, sliced

1/2 cup coconut milk

1/2 cup pineapple juice

1/2 cup ice cubes

2 tablespoons honey (optional)

1/2 teaspoon vanilla extract (optional)

Measurements:

1 cup frozen pineapple chunks

1 banana, sliced

1/2 cup coconut milk

1/2 cup pineapple juice

1/2 cup ice cubes

2 tablespoons honey (optional)

1/2 teaspoon vanilla extract (optional)

Directions:

In a blender, add the frozen pineapple chunks, sliced banana, coconut milk, pineapple juice, ice cubes, and honey (if using).

Blend until the mixture is smooth and creamy.

If desired, add in the vanilla extract and blend for a few more seconds.

Pour into glasses and serve immediately.

Nutritional Value:

This Piña Colada Smoothie is a healthy and nutritious drink that's packed with vitamins and minerals. Here's the nutritional information for one serving:

Calories: 225

Total Fat: 9g

Saturated Fat: 8g

Cholesterol: 0mg

Sodium: 11mg

Total Carbohydrates: 38g

Dietary Fiber: 3g

Sugars: 28g

Protein: 2g

Tips:

For a thicker smoothie, add more ice cubes or frozen pineapple chunks.

If you don't have pineapple juice, you can substitute with orange juice or another tropical fruit juice.

If you prefer a sweeter smoothie, add more honey or use a sweetened coconut milk.

To make the smoothie vegan, use maple syrup or agave nectar instead of honey.

If you want to make a large batch of smoothie, you can double or triple the recipe and store the extra in the fridge for later.

5. Watermelon mojito smoothie

Watermelon Mojito Smoothie is a refreshing and healthy drink that combines the sweet and juicy flavor of watermelon with the tanginess of lime and the refreshing taste of mint. Here is a recipe for making this delicious smoothie:

Ingredients:

3 cups of chopped watermelon

1/4 cup of fresh lime juice

1/4 cup of fresh mint leaves

1 cup of ice cubes

2 tbsp of honey (optional)

1/4 cup of white rum (optional)

Lime wedges and mint sprigs for garnish

Directions:

In a blender, combine the chopped watermelon, fresh lime juice, and fresh mint leaves.

Add in the ice cubes and honey (if using).

If you would like an alcoholic version of the smoothie, add in the white rum.

Blend all of the ingredients until smooth and creamy.

Pour the smoothie into glasses and garnish each glass with a lime wedge and mint sprig.

Nutritional Value:

This smoothie is a great source of vitamin C and potassium, and it is low in calories. Here is the approximate nutritional information for one serving (based on using honey instead of rum):

Calories: 84

Total Fat: 0.3g

Saturated Fat: 0g

Cholesterol: 0mg

Sodium: 2mg

Total Carbohydrates: 21g

Dietary Fiber: 1g

Sugars: 17g

Protein: 1g

Tips:

To make the smoothie even more refreshing, freeze the watermelon before blending.

If you don't have fresh lime juice, you can use bottled lime juice instead.

If you would like a sweeter smoothie, add more honey or another sweetener of your choice.

For a non-alcoholic version, simply omit the rum.

6. Spiced chai smoothie

Ingredients:

1 banana, frozen

1 cup unsweetened almond milk

1/2 cup brewed chai tea, chilled

1/4 cup rolled oats

1 tablespoon honey

1/2 teaspoon cinnamon

1/4 teaspoon ground ginger

1/8 teaspoon ground cardamom

1/8 teaspoon ground cloves

1/8 teaspoon ground nutmeg

1/2 teaspoon vanilla extract

1 cup ice cubes

Directions:

Brew a cup of chai tea and let it cool in the fridge for at least an hour before using.

In a blender, add frozen banana, almond milk, brewed chai tea, rolled oats, honey, cinnamon, ginger, cardamom, cloves, nutmeg, vanilla extract, and ice cubes.

Blend all the ingredients together until smooth and creamy.

Pour the smoothie into a glass and serve immediately.

Nutritional Information:

Serving Size: 1 smoothie

Calories: 260

Total Fat: 4g

Saturated Fat: 0.4g

Cholesterol: 0mg

Sodium: 139mg

Total Carbohydrates: 52g

Dietary Fiber: 6g

Sugars: 28g

Protein: 5g

Tips:

If you don't have a frozen banana, you can use a regular banana and add a few more ice cubes to achieve a thicker, creamier texture.

You can adjust the sweetness to your liking by adding more or less honey.

If you prefer a stronger chai flavor, you can add an extra tea bag or steep the tea for a longer time.

You can also add a scoop of protein powder to make this smoothie a complete meal.

7. Matcha madness smoothie

Ingredients:

1 banana, frozen

1 cup unsweetened almond milk

1 tsp matcha powder

1 tbsp honey or maple syrup

1 tbsp chia seeds

1/2 tsp vanilla extract

1 cup spinach

1/2 cup ice

Directions:

Begin by adding the frozen banana, unsweetened almond milk, matcha powder, honey or maple syrup, chia seeds, vanilla extract, and spinach to a blender.

Blend on high speed until the mixture is smooth and creamy.

Add the ice and continue to blend until the ice is fully incorporated and the mixture is thick and smooth.

Pour the smoothie into a glass and serve immediately.

Nutritional Information:

This matcha madness smoothie is packed with nutrients and antioxidants. Here's a breakdown of the nutritional information for one serving:

Calories: 244

Fat: 7g

Carbohydrates: 42g

Fiber: 8g

Sugar: 22g

Protein: 6g

Vitamin A: 55% DV

Vitamin C: 28% DV

Calcium: 35% DV

Iron: 16% DV

Tips:

For a creamier texture, use a frozen banana instead of a fresh one.

Add more or less honey or maple syrup to adjust the sweetness to your liking.

Use high-quality matcha powder for the best flavor and nutritional benefits.

If you don't have chia seeds, you can substitute flax seeds or omit them altogether.

If you prefer a thinner consistency, add more almond milk or water to the blender.

8. Cucumber Cooler

Ingredients:

2 medium-sized cucumbers, peeled and chopped

1 cup fresh mint leaves

1/4 cup fresh lime juice

2 tablespoons honey

4 cups cold water

Ice cubes

Optional: sliced lime and extra mint leaves for garnish.

Directions:

Add the chopped cucumbers, mint leaves, lime juice, and honey to a blender. Blend until smooth.

Pour the mixture into a large pitcher and add 4 cups of cold water. Stir to combine.

Chill the drink in the refrigerator for at least 30 minutes.

When ready to serve, add ice cubes to each glass and pour the cucumber cooler over the ice.

Optional: garnish each glass with a slice of lime and extra mint leaves.

Nutritional value:

This cucumber cooler drink is low in calories and a great source of hydration. The nutritional value of one serving (8 ounces) is approximately:

Calories: 31

Total Fat: 0 g

Sodium: 7 mg

Total Carbohydrates: 8 g

Dietary Fiber: 1 g

Sugars: 6 g

Protein: 0 g

Vitamin C: 8% of the daily value

Vitamin K: 6% of the daily value

Potassium: 4% of the daily value

Tips:

For a sweeter drink, add more honey to taste.

If you prefer a less pulpy drink, strain the mixture through a fine mesh strainer before adding water.

Make sure to chill the drink for at least 30 minutes before serving to allow the flavors to meld together.

If you don't have fresh lime juice on hand, you can use bottled lime juice instead.

This drink can be stored in the refrigerator for up to 2 days.

9. Superfood power:

Ingredients:

1 ripe banana, peeled and sliced

1 cup fresh or frozen mixed berries (such as blueberries, raspberries, and strawberries)

1/2 cup plain Greek yogurt

1/2 cup unsweetened almond milk (or any other milk of your choice)

1 tablespoon chia seeds

1 tablespoon hemp seeds

1 tablespoon ground flaxseed

1/2 teaspoon pure vanilla extract

1-2 teaspoons honey or maple syrup (optional, for sweetness)

Directions:

Add all ingredients to a blender and blend until smooth.

If the smoothie is too thick, add a little more milk to thin it out. If it's too thin, add a few ice cubes and blend again.

Taste and adjust sweetness as needed with honey or maple syrup.

Pour into a glass and enjoy!

Nutritional value:

This Superfood Power Smoothie is packed with nutrients! Here's the approximate nutritional information per serving:

Calories: 295

Fat: 11g

Carbohydrates: 37g

Fiber: 10g

Sugar: 18g

Protein: 15g

Tips:

You can use any combination of berries you like, or even just use one type if that's what you have on hand.

If you don't have chia seeds, hemp seeds, or ground flaxseed, you can use just one or two of them or substitute with another superfood like maca powder or spirulina.

If you don't have Greek yogurt, you can use any other type of plain yogurt or even silken tofu.

To make the smoothie vegan, use a non-dairy yogurt and sweeten it with maple syrup instead of honey.

If you want to make the smoothie more filling, add a scoop of protein powder or a tablespoon of nut butter.